YOUR KNOWLEDGE HAS VALUE

AF131152

- We will publish your bachelor's and master's thesis, essays and papers

- Your own eBook and book - sold worldwide in all relevant shops

- Earn money with each sale

Upload your text at www.GRIN.com and publish for free

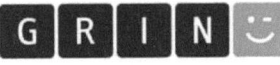

Bibliographic information published by the German National Library:

The German National Library lists this publication in the National Bibliography; detailed bibliographic data are available on the Internet at http://dnb.dnb.de .

Imprint:

Copyright © 2014 GRIN Verlag, Open Publishing GmbH
Print and binding: Books on Demand GmbH, Norderstedt Germany
ISBN: 978-3-668-04758-7

This book at GRIN:

http://www.grin.com/en/e-book/303968/studies-on-anticancer-agents-from-natural-sources-the-tabernaemontana

Manik Ghosh, Mavuduru Siva Ganesh

Studies on Anticancer Agents from Natural Sources. The Tabernaemontana Divaricata (L.) R. Br. ex Roem. & Schult.

GRIN Publishing

GRIN - Your knowledge has value

Since its foundation in 1998, GRIN has specialized in publishing academic texts by students, college teachers and other academics as e-book and printed book. The website www.grin.com is an ideal platform for presenting term papers, final papers, scientific essays, dissertations and specialist books.

Visit us on the internet:

http://www.grin.com/

http://www.facebook.com/grincom

http://www.twitter.com/grin_com

Studies on Anticancer agents from natural sources with special reference to *Tabernaemontana divaricata* (L.) R. Br. ex Roem. & Schult.

By
Dr. MANIK GHOSH
&
MAVUDURU SIVA GANESH

DEPARTMENT OF PHARMACEUTICAL SCIENCES & TECHNOLOGY
BIRLA INSTITUTE OF TECHNOLOGY
MESRA, RANCHI, INDIA-835215

CONTENTS

INTRODUCTION

CANCER

- Cancer is abnormal growth of cells generally called as malignancy.
- There are different types of cancer, ranging over 100.
- Reasons of cancer: mutation and abnormal activation of genes
- Only a small fraction of mutated genes can develop into cancer. (Guyton and Hall)
- Main reason of mutation
    - Radiations
    - Chemical irritants
    - Hereditary factors
    - Viruses

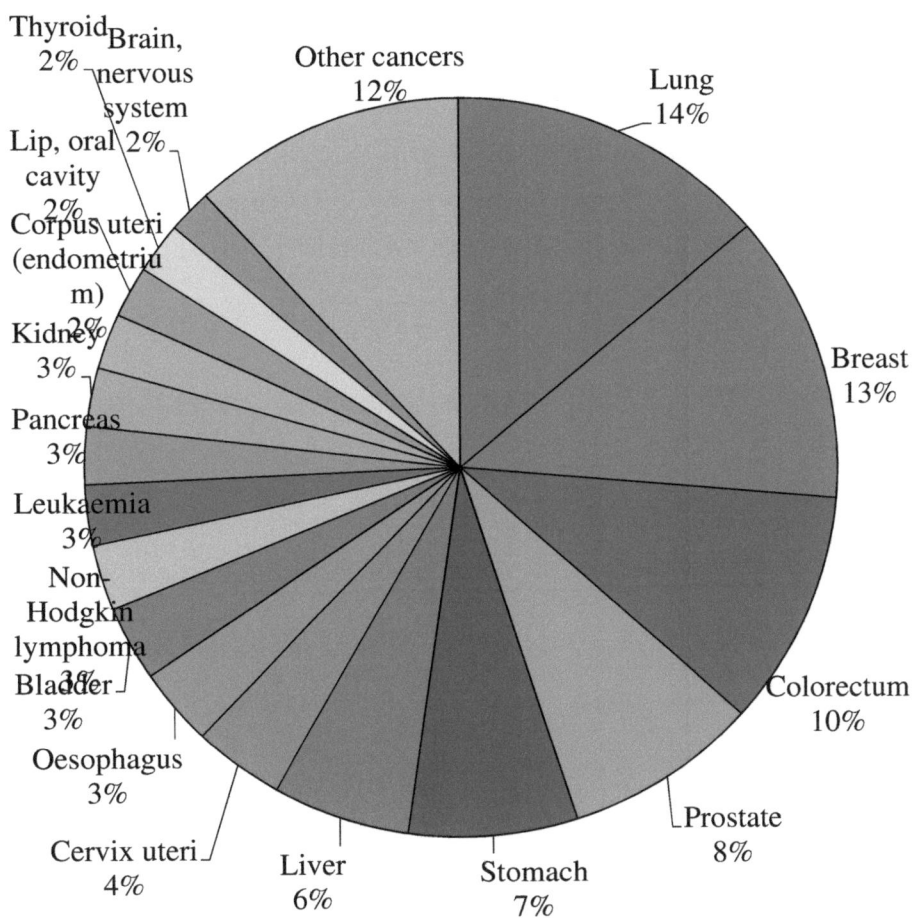

Prevalence of different types of cancer worldwide, 2012
(Source: World Cancer Research Fund International,
http://www.wcrf.org/int/cancer-facts-figures/worldwide-data)

BREAST CANCER

- Breast cancer may originate either in ducts or in glands.
- Two types: Lobular carcinoma and ductal carcinoma.
- If the cancer crosses immediate crossing, it is called invasive carcinoma (Riche and Swanson, 2003).
- Stages of breast cancer
- Stage 0- tamoxifen therapy
- Stage 1- NMT 1 inch in diameter. Not present outside breast
- Stage 2A- 1 inch
- Stage 2B- 1-2inch, may or may not spread to lymph nodes
- Stage 3A- 2 inch, spread to axillary nodes
- Stage 3B- may spread to lymph nodes attached to breast
- Stage 3C- may spread to collar bone, neck, lymph nodes in breast
- Stage 4- spread to other organs like bones, lungs and brain

ESTROGEN RECEPTOR

- Estrogens exert their activity by binding with the estrogen receptors, nuclear receptor superfamily.
- The estrogen receptor α (ERα) helps in the growth and differentiation of skeletal, neural, cardiovascular and reproductive tissues.
- ERα ligands bind mostly to the C-terminal ligand binding domain.
- Helix 12 in DES complex consists of residues from 538 to 546, in OHT complex the helix 12 consists of 536 to 544 (Shaiu et al, 1998).

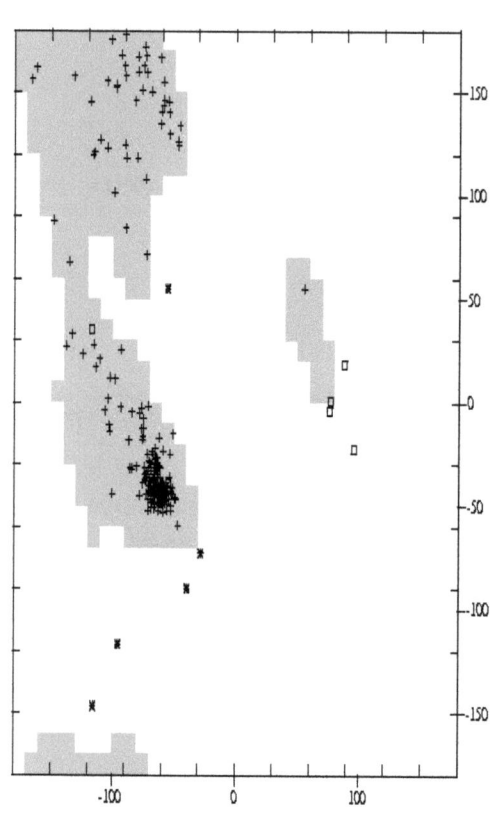

X = PHI mapped to [-180,180>

Y = PSI mapped to [-180,180>

PDB file : /pub/db/pub/pdb/data/structures/all/pdb/pdb3ert.ent

Glycines (open squares): 10 ; Start/end residues : 2

D-amino acids : 0 ; Residues with missing atoms : 1

Residues in Ramachandran plot checked : 234 out of 247

In core regions (plus signs): 229 ; Outliers (asterisks): 5

Percentage outliers: 2.1

An average <= 2.0 A model has ~0-5% outliers

See: Kleywegt, G.J. and Jones, T.A. (1996). Structure 4, 1395-1400.

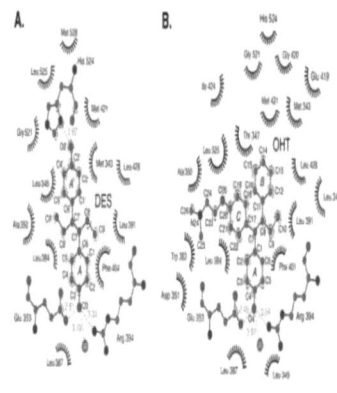

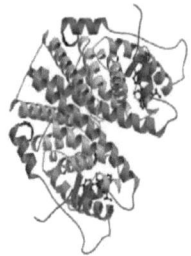

ESTROGEN RECEPTOR

Source: http://www.rcsb.org/pdb/images/1sj0_bio_r_500.jpg

RAMCHANDRAN PLOT

Reproduced from: www.rcsb.org

8

MCF-7 CELL LINE

○ Isolated from 69 year old Caucasian woman's cancer cells

○ Malignant adenocarcinoma in a pleural effusion was removed in the second surgery, from which MCF-7 cell lines were prepared.

○ Initially 85 karyotypes in the chromosomes. Later it was reduced to 69.

○ Characteristics: sensitive to cytokeratin, Tumor necrosis factor alpha (TNF alpha) can inhibit growth.

Desmin, endothelin, and vimentin are unresponsive to

MCF-7 cell line

(www.mcf7.com).

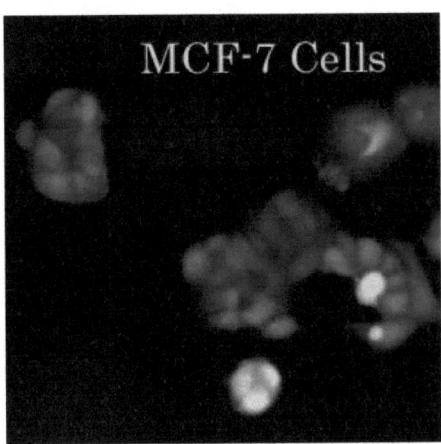 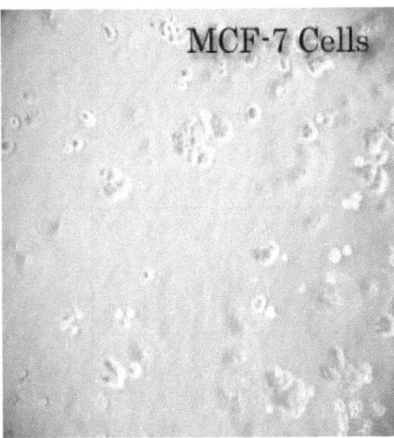

Reproduced from:

TABERNAEMONTANA DIVARICATA

KINGDOM:	Plantae
ORDER:	Gentianales
FAMILY:	Apocynaceae
SUBFAMILY:	Rauvolfioideae
GENUS:	*Tabernaemontana*
SPECIES:	*divaricata*

Alkaloids	Medicinal activity
12-hydroxy akuammicine	Raise in tone/frequency of rabbit uterus
19,20-dihydrotabernamine	Inhibit Acetylcholine esterase
Catharanthine	Differentiation of pancreatic tumor cells.
Coronaridine	Analgesic and anti-inflammatory effect

LITERATURE REVIEW

LITERATURE: ANTICANCER PLANTS

○ **Masfria et al. (2013)** -anticancer properties of ethanolic extract of *Rhaphidophora pinnta.*

○ **Valiyari et al. (2013)** -anticancer and cyctotoxic activity of *Scrophularia oxysepala.*

  ⦾ The dichloromethane and methanol extract found to have the cytotoxic activity.

  ⦾ Reason- induction of apotosis

○ **Elkady et al. (2012)** -anticancer properties of *Zingiber officinale.*

  ⦾ Methanolic extract was having antiproliferative effect.

○ **Kundu et al. (2012)**- antimetastatic property of *Colocasia esculenta.* Water extracts of the plant showed significant antimetastatic property in tumor induced mammary glands.

○ **Sepehr et al. (2011)**- anticancer effect of extracts from *Cuscuta kotschyana* on MCF 7 cell line. The flavonoids extracts were tested for anticancer properties.

○ **Duarte et al. (2010)** - isolated two alkaloids from *Pterogyne nitens,* namely pterogynine and pterogynidine tested for infiltrating ductal carcinoma cell line.

  ⦾ They found that both the alkaloids have significant anticancer properties by inducing programmed cell death.

- **Orawan et al. (2005)-** isolated belalloside A, belalloside B, and belamphenone and thirteen known compounds from the rhizomes of *Belamcanda chinensis*. Belamphenone was found to stimulate MCF-7 cell lines.

- **Lee et al. (2003)-** isolated styrylpyrone derivative from *Goniothalamus* species showed antiproliferative activity using MCF-7 cell line.
  - Reason: regulation of Bax protein expression

- **Julio et al. (2000)-** isolated glycoconjugate from *Crocus sativus*.
  - The compound showed an IC_{50} value of 22µg/ml when tested for anticancer activity against breast cancer using MCF-7 cell line.

- **Surendra et al. (1997)** has found that curcumin and genistein has synergitic activity on antiproliferative effect of human breast cancer cell line (MCF-7).

- **Scambia et al. (1994)-**quercetin elevates the activity of Adiramycin in multi-drug resistant breast cancer using MCF-7 cell line.

LITERATURE REVIEW
Tabernaemontana divaricata

○ **Chaiyana et al. (2013)-** isolated 3'-R/S-hydroxyvoacamine, a potent acetylcholinesterase inhibitor from the stem of *Tabernaemontana divaricata*. The alkaloid acted as non-competitive inhibitor of AChE and has IC_{50} value of 7.00 ± 1.99µM.

○ **Bao et al. (2013)-** isolated five novel vobasinyl-ibogan-type bisindole alkaloids.

- named as tabernaricatines A-E. They have extracted 24 known indole alkaloids, among them; conophylline gave significant anticancer activities with IC_{50} values of 0.17, 0.35, 0.21, 1.02, and 1.49µM on HL-60, SMMC-7721, A-549, MCF-7, and SW480 cell lines respectively.

○ **Mukhram et al. (2012)-** established the anti-fertility property of *Tabernaemontana divaricata* flower extracts in rats.

- The extracts were obtained using methanol and water. The anti-fertility effects were studied using estrogenic activity, anti-implantation and early abortifacient effect.
- methanolic extract of *Tabernaemontana divaricata* at at 500mġ kg^{-1}, has estrogenic, anti-implantation and abortifacient activity.

- **Raj and Balasubramaniam (2011)-** studied the antimicrobial properties of *Tabernaemontana divaricata.*
  - The extracts were obtained using petroleum ether, chloroform, methanol and water. Tested against gram positive and negative bacteria
  - Had moderate activity on both the bacteria.
- **Kam et al. (2004)** have isolated five new indole alkaloids namely (3S)-3-cyanocoronaridine,(3S)-3-cyanoisovoacangine, conolobine A, conolobine B, conolidine, and (3R/3S)-3-ethoxyvoacangine.
- **Keimei et al. (1998)-** isolated conophylline from *Tabernaemontana divaricata.*
- **Arambewela and Ranatunge (1991)-** isolated eleven indole alkaloids namely voacangine, voacristine, isovoacristine, coronaridine, isovoacangine, vobasine, voacangine, tabernaemontanine, 19-epi-voacangine from the leaves of *Tabernaemontana divaricata.*

Conophylline

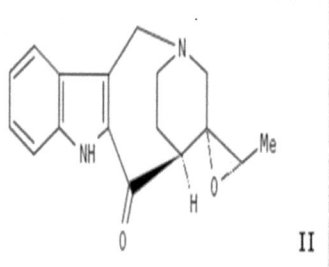

Conolobine A

II

Conolobine B

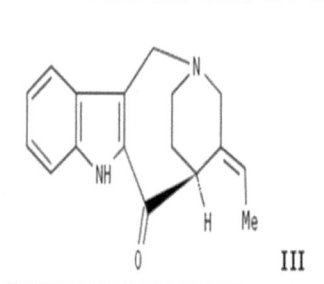

III

Conolidine

Tabernaemontanine

19-epi voacangine

Isovocangine

OBJECTIVES AND PLAN OF WORK

OBJECTIVES

- Breast cancer is the most prevalent cancer in women. Currently the drugs available for breast cancer have a disadvantage of having severe adverse effects and decreasing the quality of life.

- Guided by the literature review and followed by docking studies of phytoconstituents it was found worthy to scientifically explore Tabernaemontana divaricata w.r.t its phytochemical presence and anticancer activities.

- In the present study, the main aim was to identify the most potent extract against breast cancer from leaves of Tabernaemontana divaricata (L.) R. Br. ex Roem. & Schult.

- From the most potent extract, we aim to isolate the phytoconstituents and to test their efficacy against breast cancer.

-

- Further docking studies need to be performed, to know the docking poses of known phytoconstituents.

- Antioxidant studies and toxicity studies need to be performed to assess the pharmacological activities of plant extract and isolated compounds.

EXPERIMETAL WORK

DOCKING STUDIES

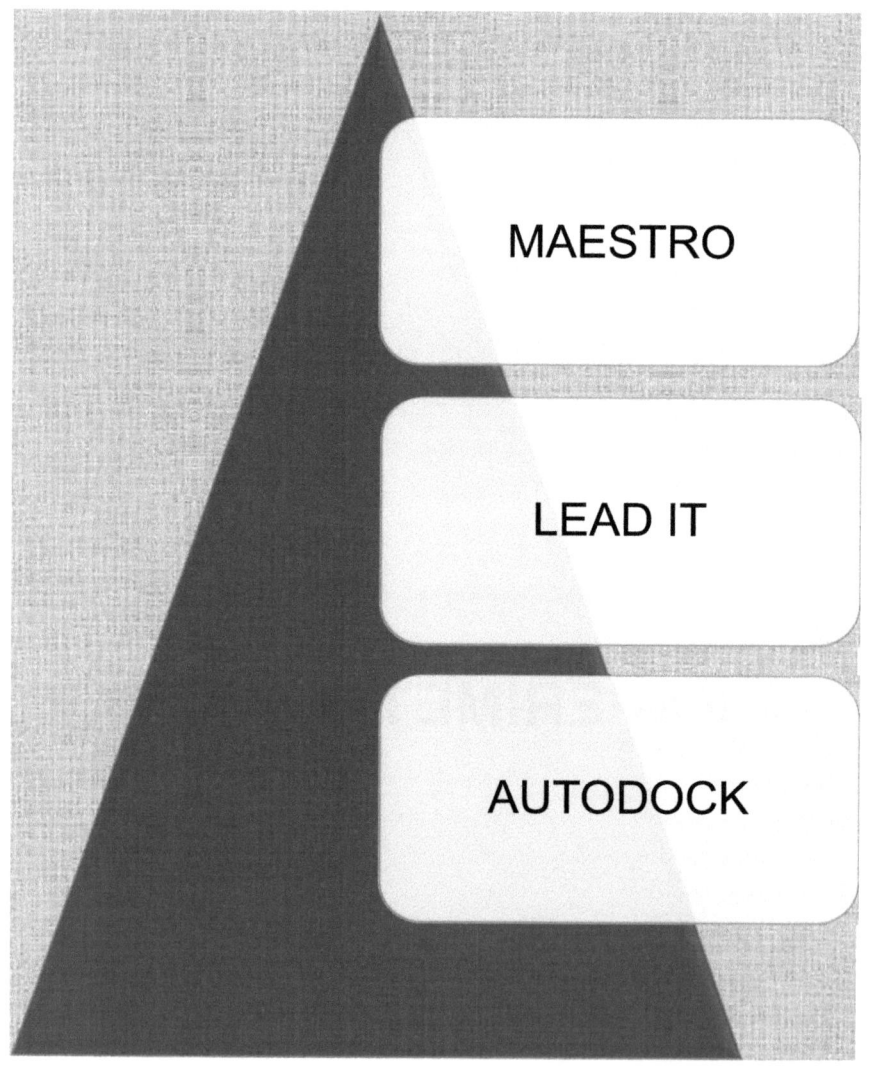

MAESTRO

PROTEIN PREPARATION: 3ERT was processed, Water molecules- deleted. Hydrogen, disulphide bonds- added. Heterostates were generated. Energy minimized using OPLS 2001 force field.

LIGAND PREPARATION: Force filed used was OPLS_2001.

All possible heterostates were generated. All possible stereoisomers were generated.

RECEPTOR GRID GENERATION & LIGAND DOCKING: Co-crystallized molecule was selected as grid center and docking was performed using Standard Precision

LEADIT

Protein preparation: Particular chains were selected as receptor, binding site was defined and chemical ambiguities were resolved.

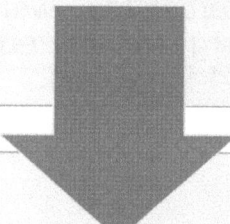

Ligand preparation

Prepared in maestro were used in .sdf format

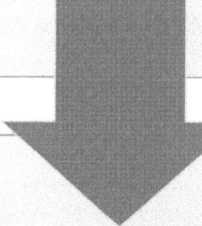

Docking: Performed used hybrid approach

Protein preparation: Prepared
in maestro was converted into
Autodock compatible type

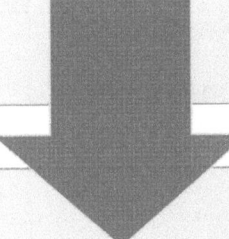

Ligand preparation

Prepared in maestro was converted
into Autodock compatible type

Grid generation: Grid parameter file
(.gpf) & drug parameter file (.dpf)
were generated using MGL Tools-
1.4.6.

Docking: Runs: 50, population size:
150, number of evaluations
2500000 and generations: 27000.

DOCKING STUDIES

Standard compounds	Scores			
	Maestro	Lead IT	Autodock	
	Docking score		Free binding energy	Estimated inhibition constant
4-hydroxy tamoxifen	-11.28	-34.94	-4.18	859.08µM
Doxorubicin	-6.10	-17.67	-7.38	30.73µM
Dreganine	-6.03	-13.62	-4.38	598.09µM
Catharanthine	-6.32	-20.79	7.72	6.06µM
Taebernaemonta nine	-3.69	-20.03	-7.53	2.20µM
Conophylline	ND	ND	-3.76	824.58µM

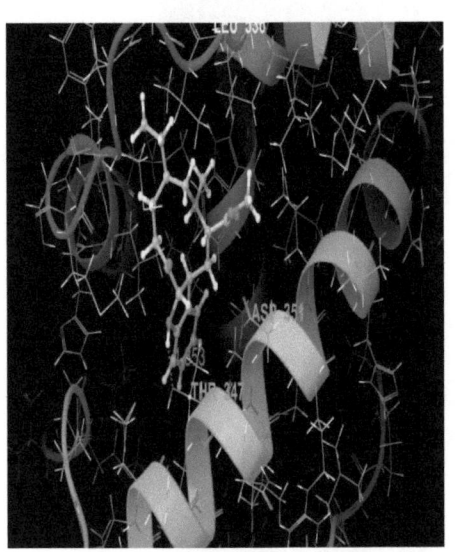 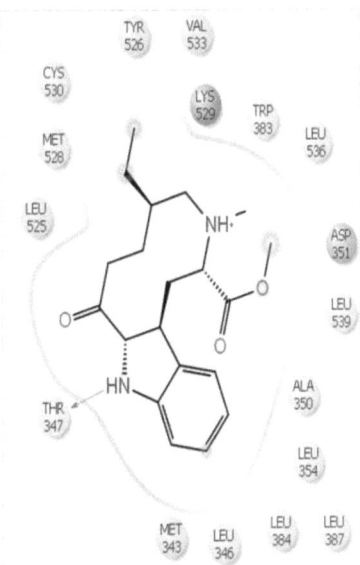

Interaction of dreganine with 3ERT in maestro forming H-bond with Thr 347 of length 1.853Å

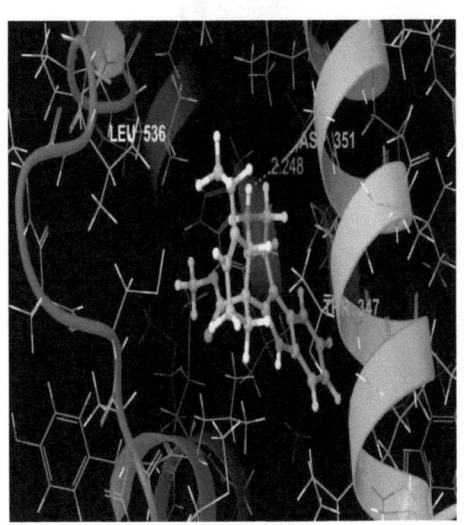 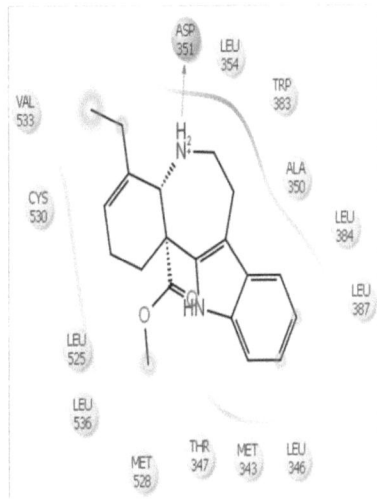

Interaction of catharanthine with 3ERT in maestro forming H-bond with Asp 351 of length 2.248Å

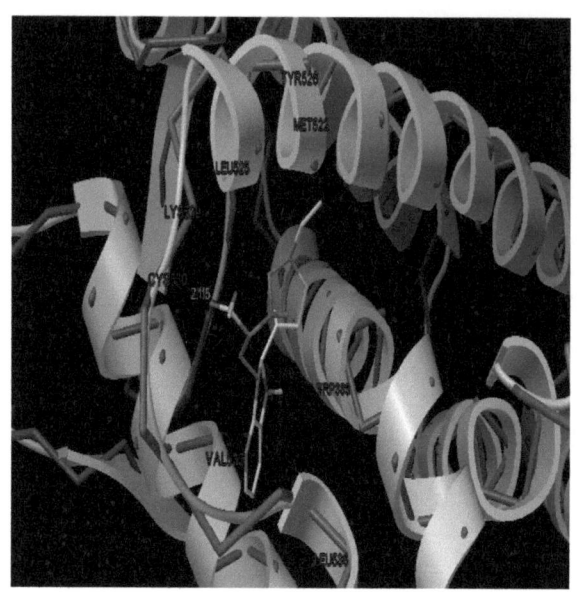

Docking pose of Dreganine interacting with Cys 530 with H-bond length of 2.115Å

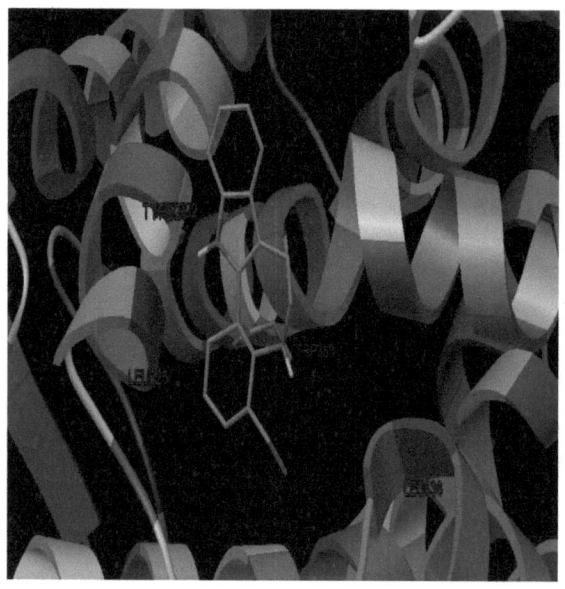

Docking pose of Catharanthine

PHYTOCHEMICAL STUDIES

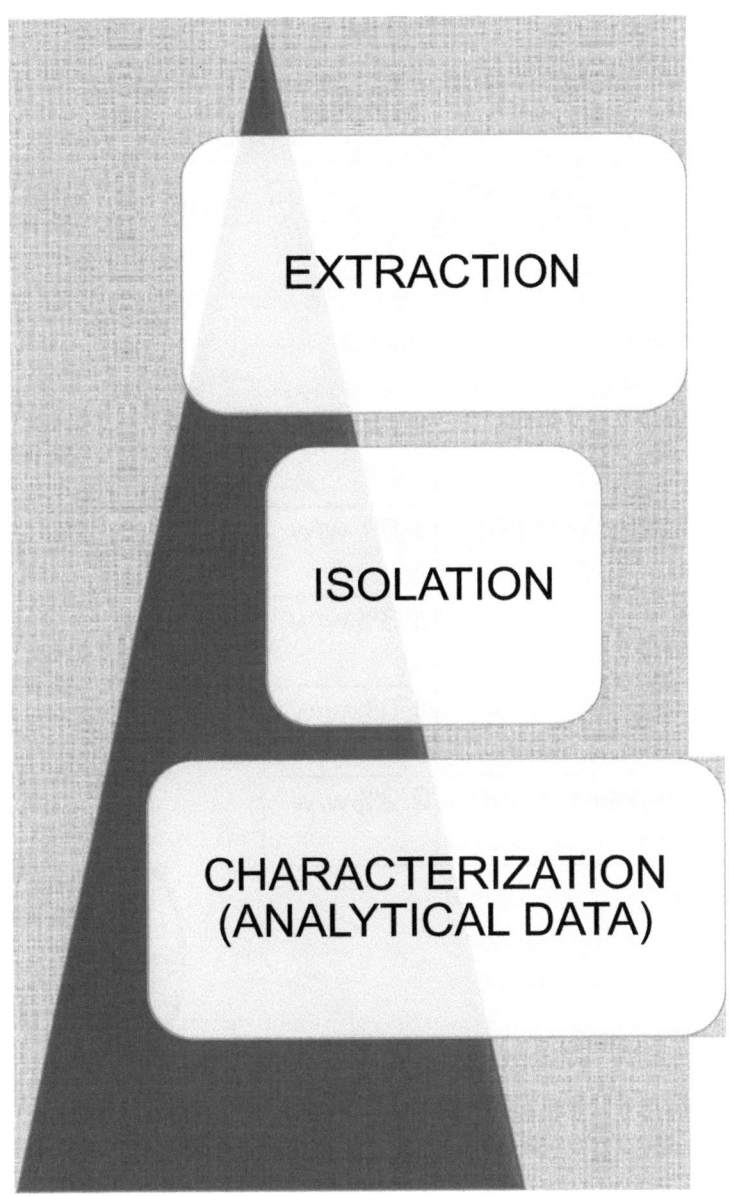

EXTRACTION

* Defating for 72 hrs using Petroleum ether (60-80 °C)

* Successive extraction using chloroform, ethyl acetate, 80%v/v methanol for 48 hours.

* Extractive values

1	Petroleum ether (60-80)	1.6%w/w
2	Chloroform	1.3%w/w
3	Ethyl acetate	1.0%w/w
4	Methanol : water (80:20)	2.2%w/w

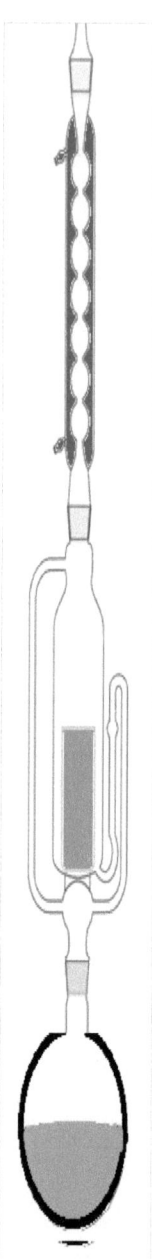

PHYTOCHEMICAL SCREENING

TEST	RESULT AND INFERENCE

TEST FOR ALKALOIDS

A)Dragendorff's Reagent	Reddish brown precipitate
B)Wagner's reagent	Reddish brown precipitate
C)Hager's reagent	Buff coloured precipitate

TEST FOR FLAVONOIDS

A) Shinoda's test	Red colour
B) Alkaline reagent test	Yellow colour turns to colourless on addition of acid

TEST	RESULT AND INFERENCE

TEST FOR GLYCOSIDES

A) Borntrager's test	Rose pink colour
B) Keller Kiliani test	Bluish green layer of acetic acid
C) Legal test	Pink colour

TEST FOR STEROIDS

A) Libermann-Burchard test	Red colour at junction
B) Salkowski test	Yellow colour

TEST	RESULT AND INFERENCE

TEST FOR TANNINS

A) Ferric chloride test	Blue colour in case of hydrolysable tannins and green colour in case of condensed tannins
B) Extract + potassium dichromate	Brown precipitate

PHYTOCHEMICAL SCREENING

Phytoconstituents	Pet. ether	Chloroform	Ethyl Acetate	80% Methanol
Alkaloids	-	-	+	+
Flavonoids	-	-	+	+
Steroids & triterpenes	+	+	-	-
Carbohydrates	-	-	+	+
Saponins	-	-	-	-
Glycosides	-	+	+	+
Tannins	-	-	+	+

ISOLATION

- **TLC STUDIES**
- Solvent system: Petroleum ether: n-hexane: toluene: ethyl acetate in the ratio 3:3:1:2.5

- **HPTLC STUDIES:** Performed using Linomat IV, Camag TLC scanner and Cats 4.0 software.
- Material of HPTLC plates: Silica gel 60 F_{254}
- Plate size (X x Y)   :5.0 x 10.0 cm
- Number of tracks   :2
- Position of first track X   12.0 mm
- Distance between tracks   12.0 mm;.
- Scan start pos. Y: 12.5 mm
- Scan end pos. Y   :80.0 mm

PHYTOCHEMICAL STUDIES

HPTLC studies

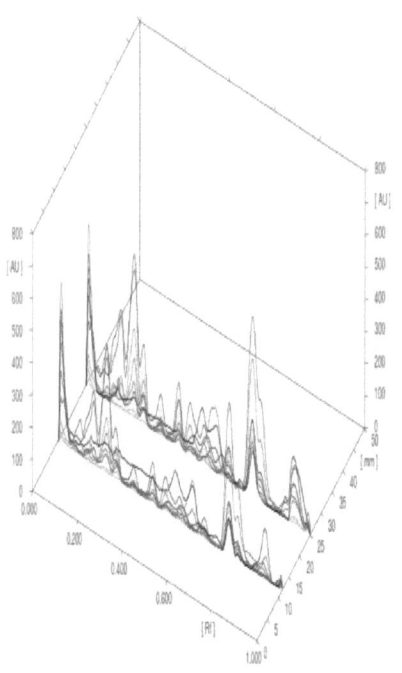

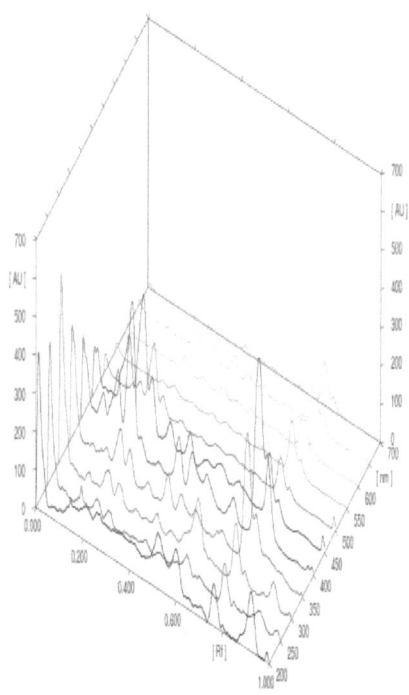

Peaks indicating the separation of compounds

Peaks indicating the separation of compounds at different wavelengths

COLUMN CHROMATOGRAPHY

2 phytochemicals were isolated with Rf of 0.9 and 0.2

Wet column prepared using 100-200 column grade Silica gel

Extraction for several times

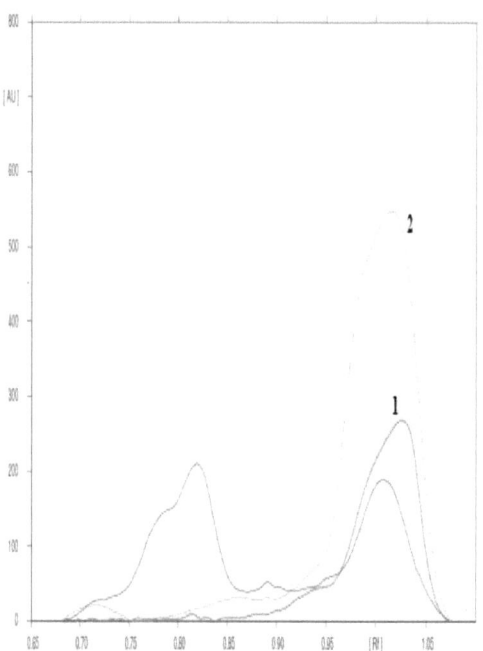

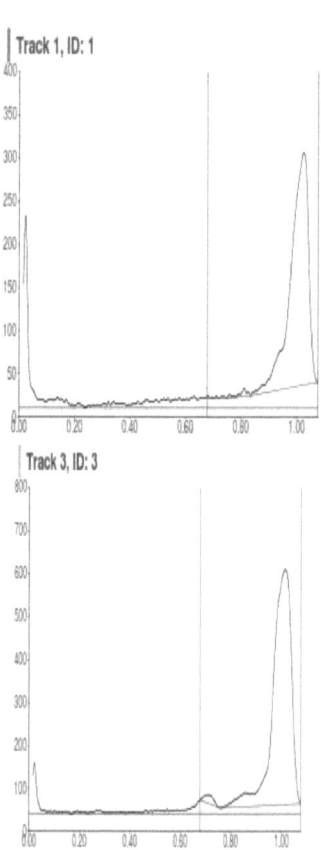

HPTLC of two compounds, 1-Compound 1, 2- Compound 2; B-HPTLC of compound 1 and C-HPTLC of compound 2

ANALYTICAL DATA

UV-Visibile spectroscopy	• Absorption maxima was determining at a concentration of 5µg/ml
FT-IR	• 1mg compound + 100 mg KBR – to determine functional groups
^{1}NMR	•Obtained at 400 MHz in $CDCl_3$ using a Varian 400 (Varian Inc., USA).
MS	• Using WATERS-Q-T of Premier-HAB213.

SPECTRAL STUDIES OF COMPOUND 1

UV-Visible spectroscopy (in chloroform)

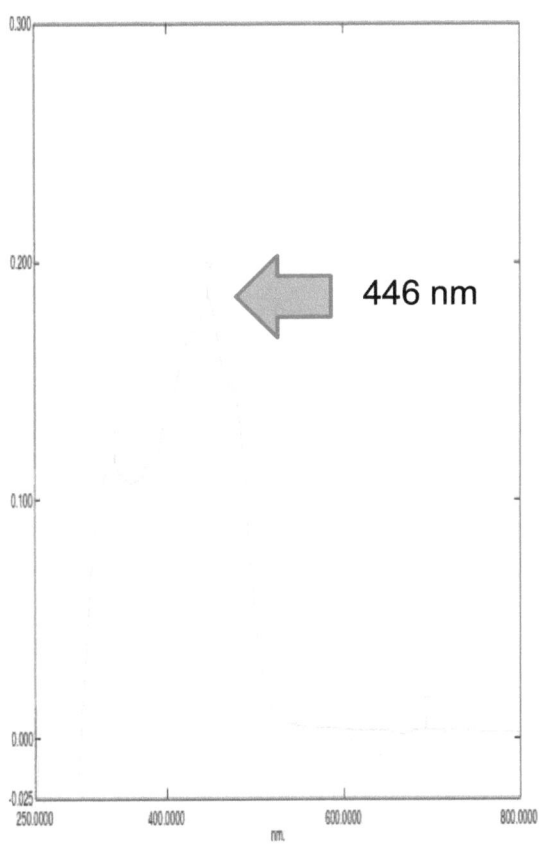

446 nm

Absorption maximum

446 nm

FT-IR OF COMPOUND 1 (USING POTASSIUM BROMIDE)

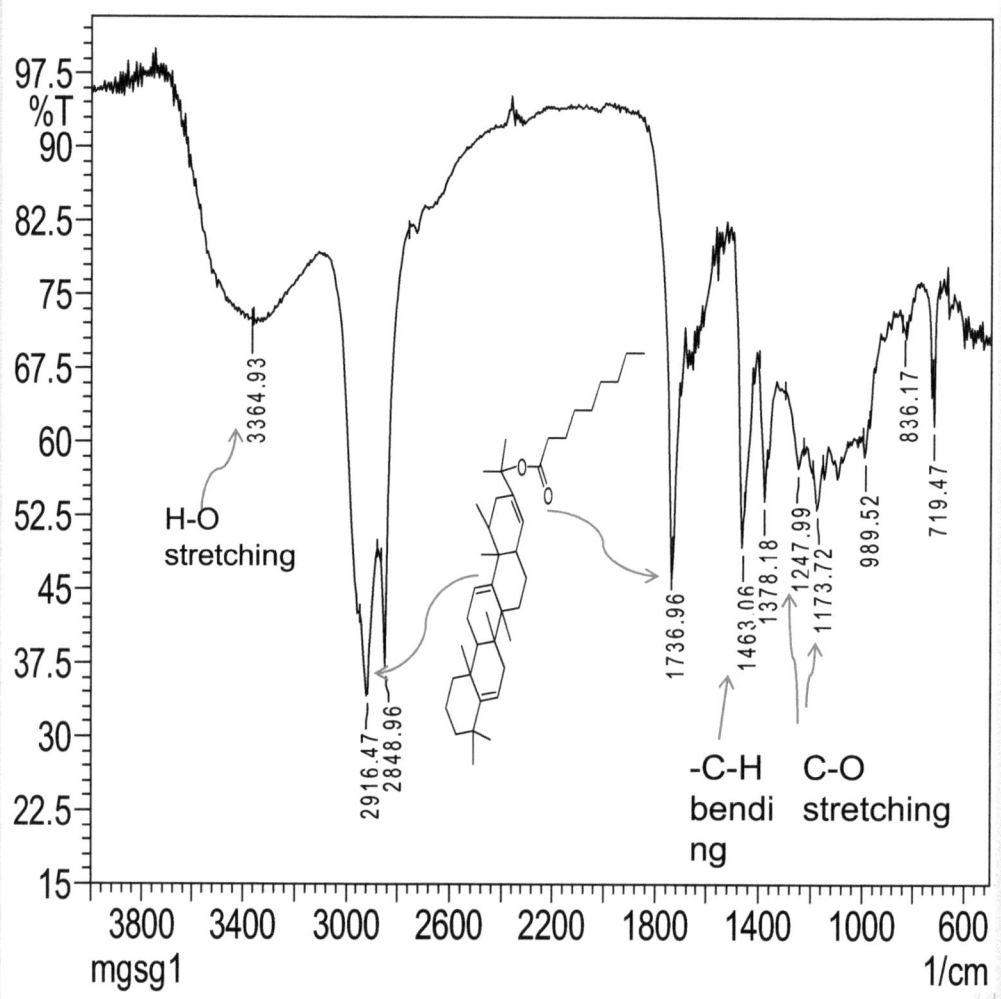

¹H NMR SPECTRA OF COMPOUND 1

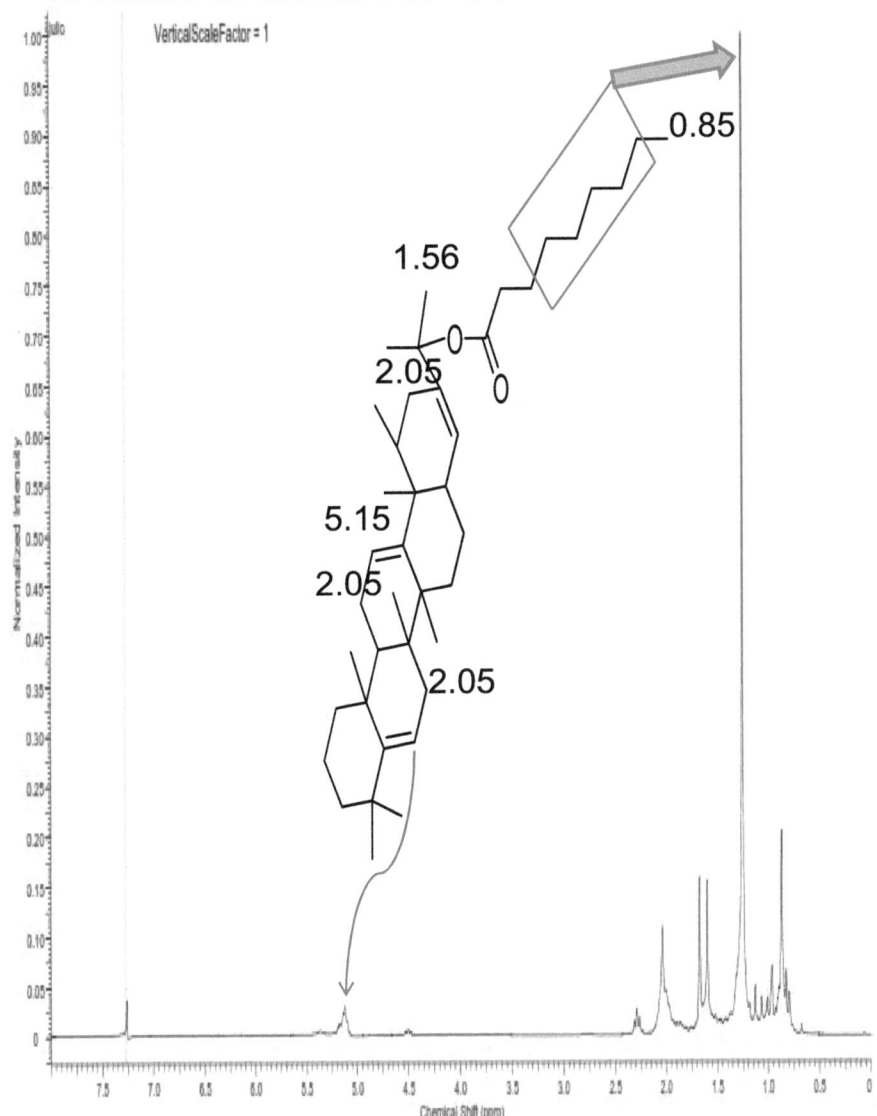

VerticalScaleFactor = 1

1.56

2.05

5.15

2.05

2.05

0.85

Normalized Intensity

Chemical Shift (ppm)

MASS SPECTRA OF COMPOUND 1

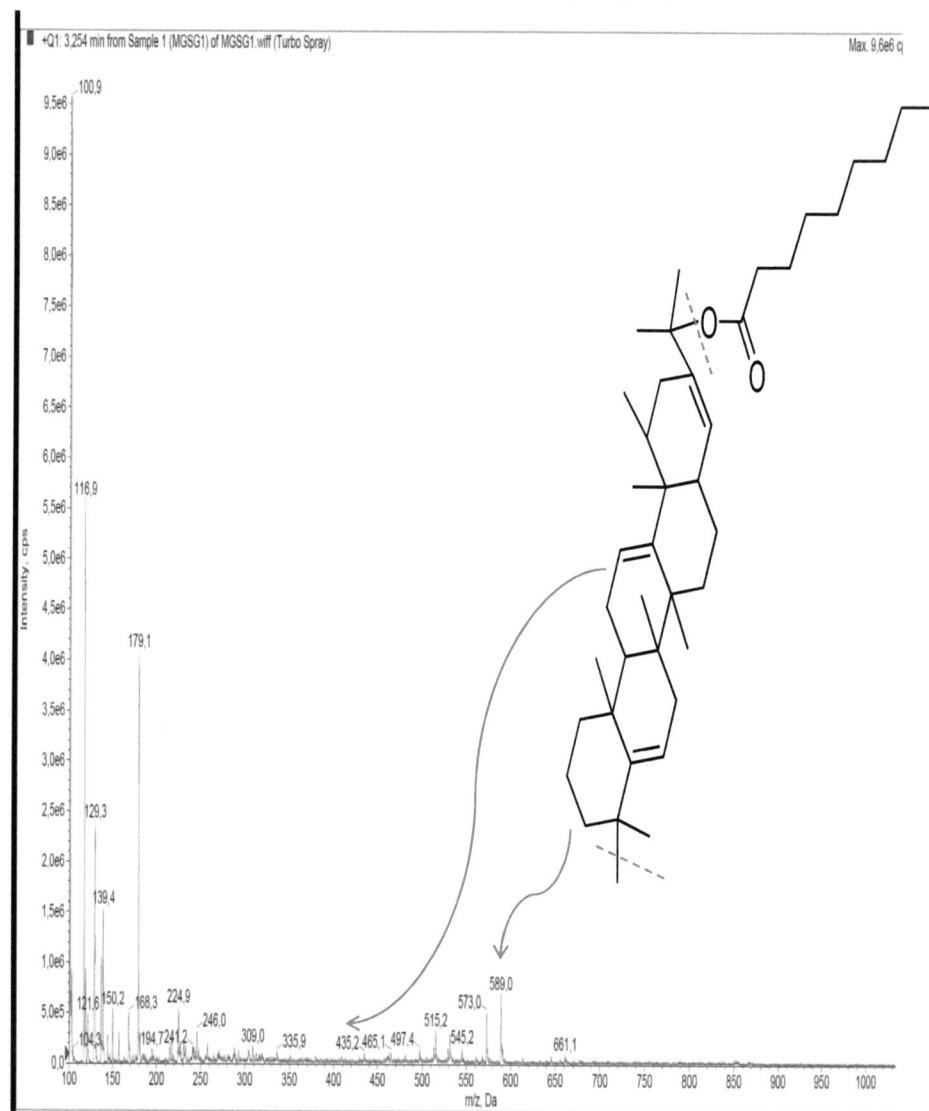

STRUCTURE OF COMPOUND 1

Melting point   :140-142 $^\circ$ C

UV (nm)   :446

FT-IR (cm^{-1})   :
3364.93, 2916.47, 2848.96, 1736.96,
1463.06, 1378.18, 1247.99, 1173.72,
989.52, 836.17, 719.47

ESI-MS (m/z)   : 589

^{1}H *NMR* (δ ppm) :
0.68, 0.80, 0.87, 0.97, 1.0,
1.15, 1.3, 1.6, 1.68, 2.1,
2.3, 4.5, 5.15

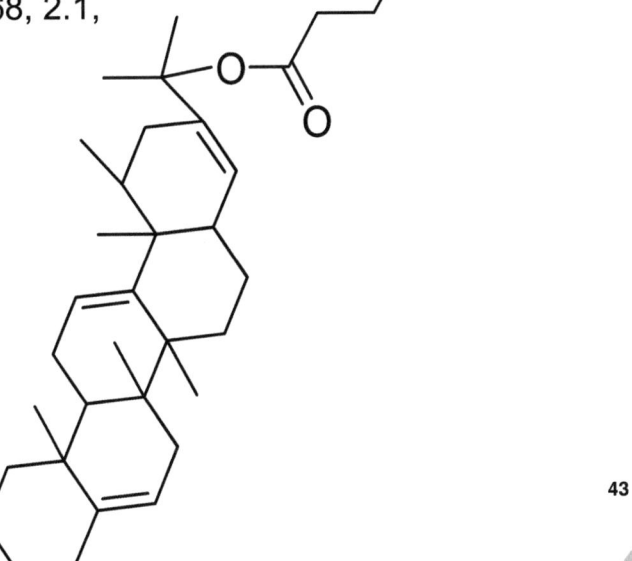

SPECTRAL DATA OF COMPOUND 2

UV-VISIBLE SPECTROSCOPY OF COMPOUND 2

- Absorption maxima
    447nm

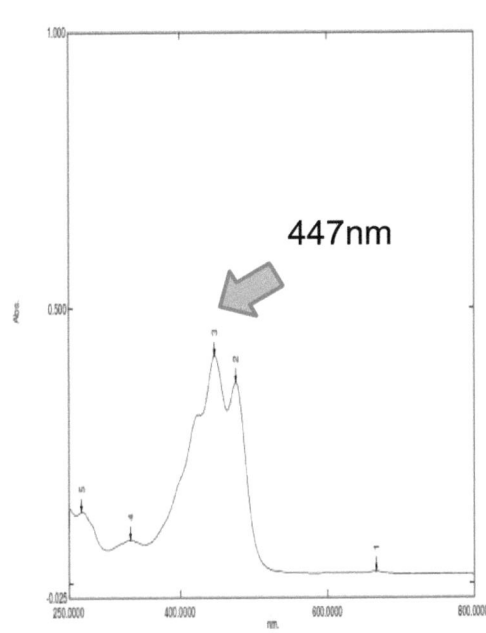

FT-IR OF COMPOUND 2

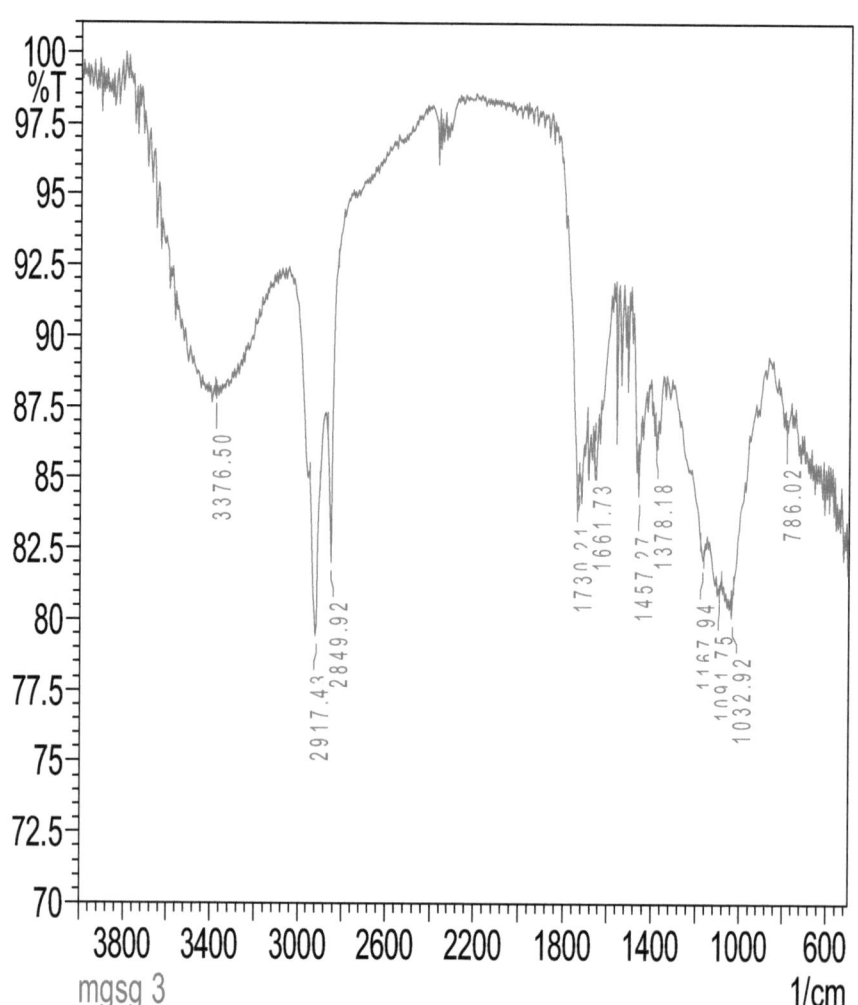

mgsg 3

1/cm

¹H NMR OF COMPOUND 2

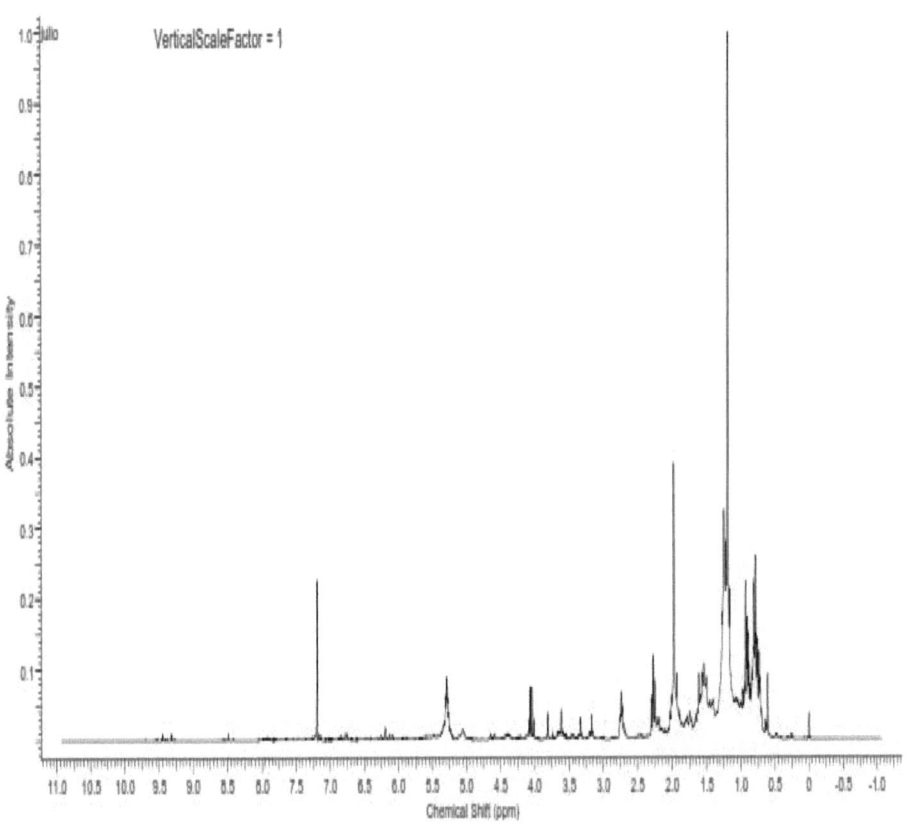

Ms OF COMPOUND 2

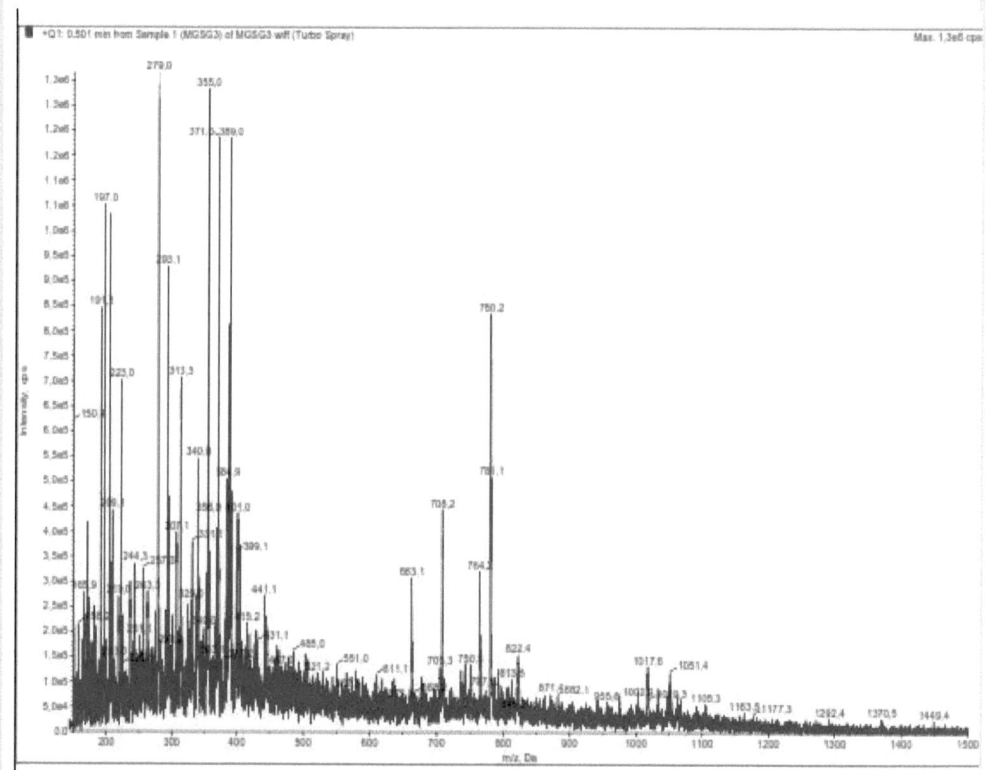

PHARMACOLOGICAL STUDIES

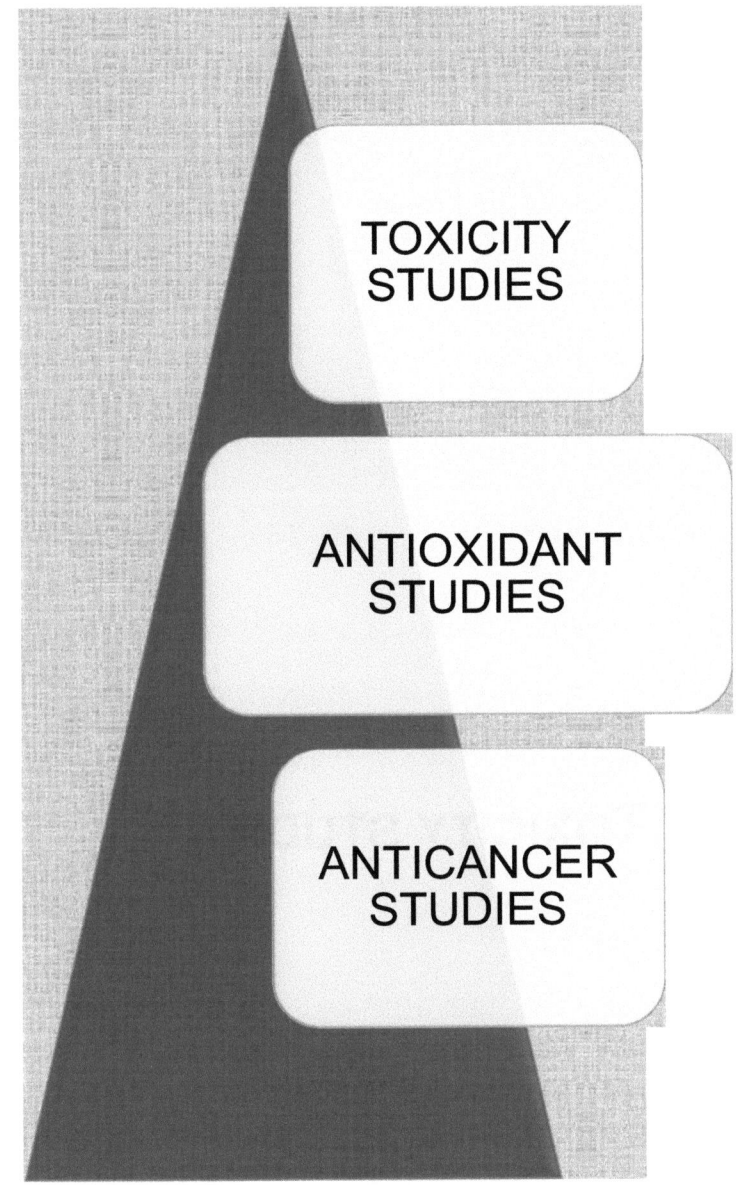

TOXICITY
STUDIES

ANTIOXIDANT
STUDIES

ANTICANCER
STUDIES

TOXICITY STUDIES

TOXICITY STUDIES

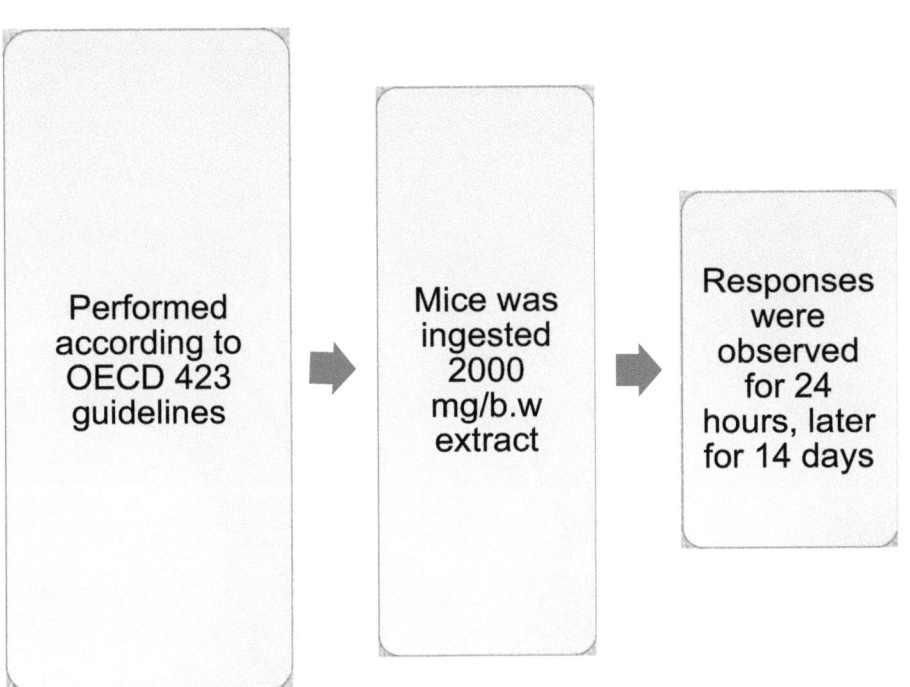

Performed according to OECD 423 guidelines → Mice was ingested 2000 mg/b.w extract → Responses were observed for 24 hours, later for 14 days

Test substance	Dose	Mortality rate
Petroleum ether extract of *Tabernaemontana divaricata*	2000 mg/kg b.w	Nil

ANTI OXIDANT STUDIES

ANTIOXIDANT STUDIES
DPPH ASSAY

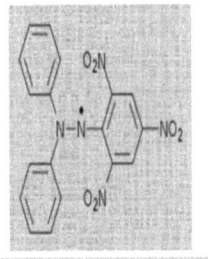 DPPH

20, 50, 100, 200, 500 and 1000 µg/ml solutions of compounds were prepared. 40, 80, 120, 160, 200 µg/ml were selected for further studies

Sample- 1ml sample + 2ml DPPH solution

Control- 1ml methanol+ 2ml DPPH solution

Absorbance was taken at 517nm. Ascorbic acid was used as standard.

$$Scavenging\ activity\ (\%) = 1 - \frac{absorbance\ of\ sample}{absorbance\ of\ control} \times 100$$

ANTIOXIDANT STUDIES

Anti-oxidant activity of standard (ascorbic acid)

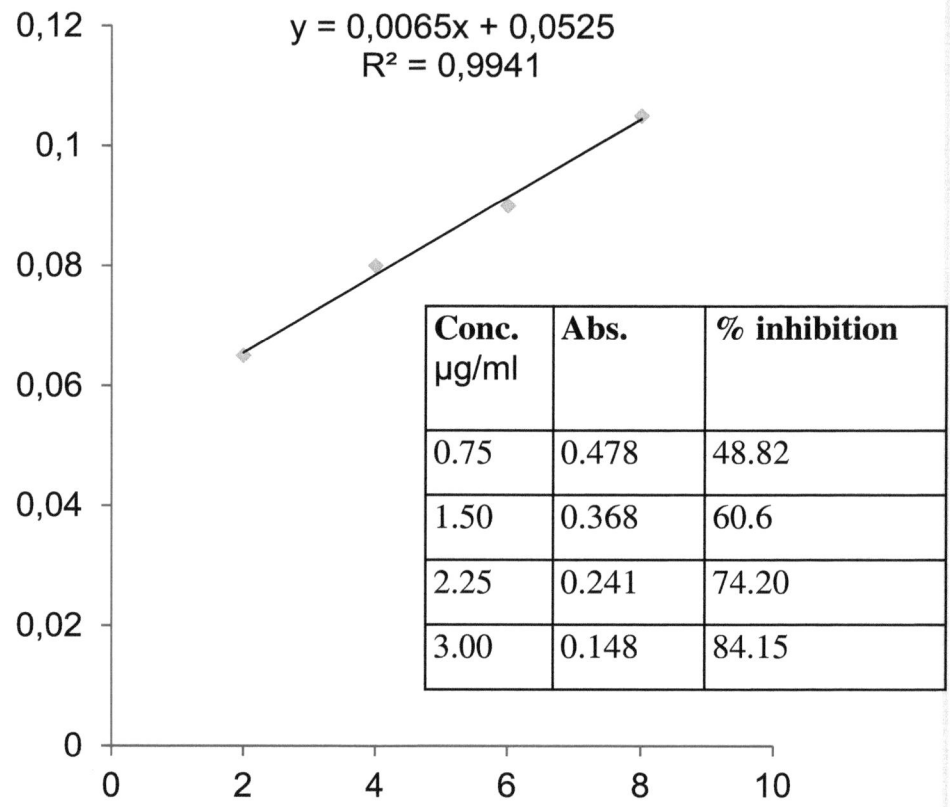

$y = 0,0065x + 0,0525$
$R^2 = 0,9941$

Conc. µg/ml	Abs.	% inhibition
0.75	0.478	48.82
1.50	0.368	60.6
2.25	0.241	74.20
3.00	0.148	84.15

Anti-oxidant assay of standard (ascorbic acid)

The IC_{50} value was found to be 0.81µg/ml.

Anti-oxidant studies of petroleum ether extract and compounds

Sample	*Tabernaemontana divaricata* petroleum ether extract		Compound 1		Compound 2	
Conc. µg/ml	Abs	Percent inhibition	Abs	Percent inhibition	Abs	Percent inhibition
40	0.904	3.21	0.808	13.49	0.784	16.06
80	0.816	12.63	0.626	32.98	0.604	35.33
120	0.704	24.63	0.528	43.47	0.498	46.68
160	0.6021	35.55	0.324	65.31	0.298	68.09
200	0.514	44.97	0.258	72.38	0.218	76.67

IC_{50} value of petroleum ether extract   217µg/ml
IC_{50} value of compound 1   132.08µg/ml
IC_{50} value of compound 2   128.90µg/ml

ANTICANCER STUDIES

Growth medium

- RPMI 1640 growth medium + 10% fetal bovine serum + 2mM L-glutamine

Culture conditions

- 37° C in a humidified atmosphere of 5% CO_2.

Cell proliferation studies

- Plate seeded with 5 x 10^3 cells fixed with TCA

- Testing sample + dimethyl sulfoxide at 100mg/ml conc

- diluted to 1mg/ml conc

- Serial dilutions: 100µg/ml, 200µg/ml, 400µg/ml and 800µg/ml

- 10µl from each dilution to 90µl of the medium resulting in the concentration of 10 µg/ml, 20µg/ml, 40 µg/ml and 80µg/ml.

Anticancer assay using MCF-7 cell line

SRB assay method

- Satining : 0.4% (w/v) Sulforhodamine B (SRB) solution in 1% acetic acid

- Washing: acetic acid

- optical density (OD) bound dye was solubilized with 10mM Tris [tris (hydroxymethyl)aminomethane] base for 5 minutes on a gyratory shaker

- OD determined at 564nm

$$Percentage\ growth = \frac{Absorbance\ of\ control\ wells}{Average\ absorbance} \times 100$$

$$\%\ of\ control\ cell\ growth = \frac{mean\ OD\ sample - mean\ OD\ day\ 0}{mean\ OD\ negative\ control - mean\ OD\ day\ 0} \times 100$$

ANTICANCER STUDIES

Anticancer studies extracts and isolated compounds from
Tabernaemontana divaricata **(Concentrations in μg/ml)**

Extracts	10	20	40	80	LC50	TGI	GI50
Pet. ether extract	31.2	29.5	27.4	26.0	>80	>80	18.7
Chloroform extract	91.6	87.3	69.2	49.4	>80	>80	77.4
Ethyl acetate extract	97.3	97.0	89.5	74.9	>80	>80	>80
Isolated	**10**	**20**	**40**	**80**	**LC50**	**TGI**	**GI50**
Compound 1	100	98.3	94.3	87.6	>80	>80	>80
Compound 2	90.1	85.0	77.0	59.1	>80	>80	>80
Standard	**10**	**20**	**40**	**80**	**LC50**	**TGI**	**GI50**
Adiramycin	3.5	-1.8	-8.9	-30.7	>80	41.6	<10

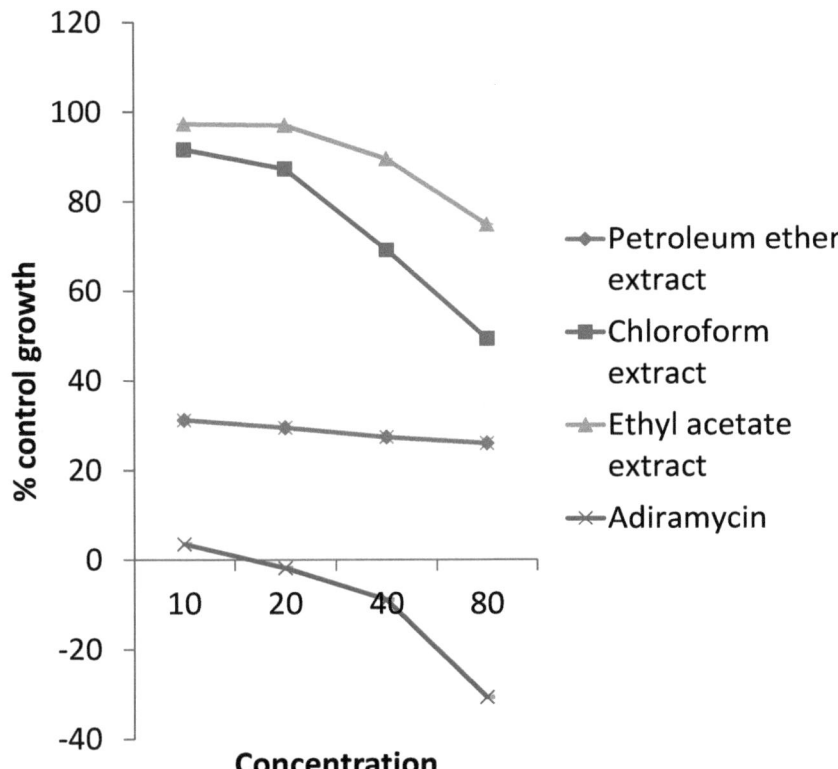

Growth Curve: Human Breast Cancer Cell Line MCF7 of three different extract of *Tabernaemontana divaricata*

GI_{50} value of petroleum ether extract :   18.7 µg/ml

GI_{50} value of chloroform extract :   77.4 µg/ml

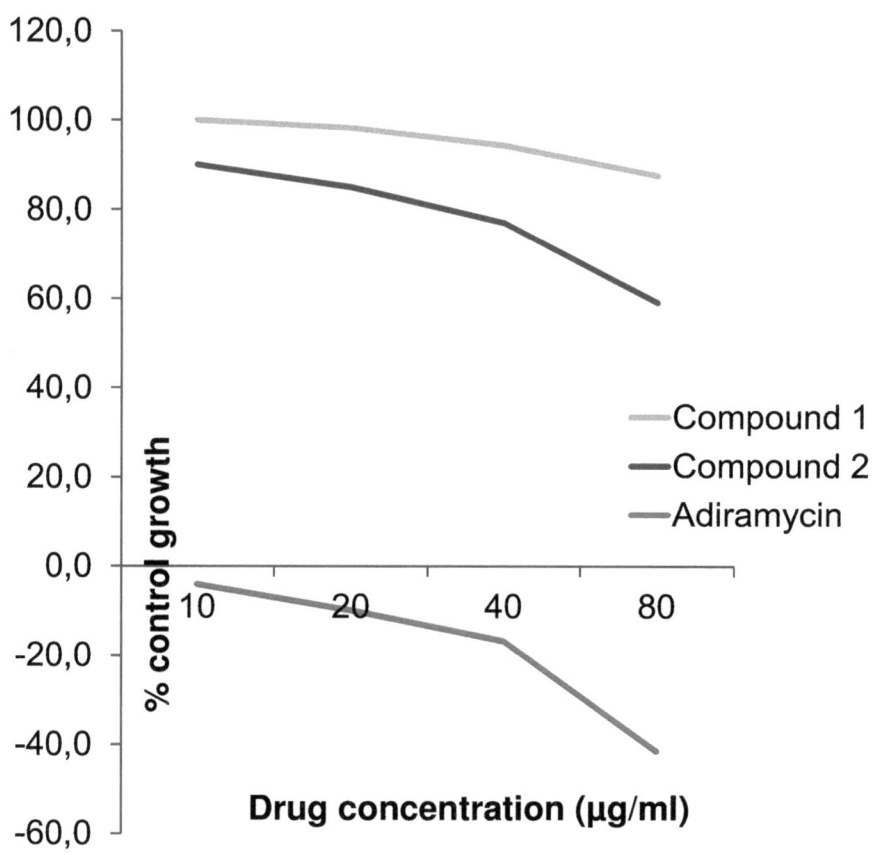

Growth Curve: Human Breast Cancer Cell Line MCF7 of three different extract of *Tabernaemontana divaricata*

GI_{50} value of petroleum ether extract   >80

GI_{50} value of chloroform extract   >80

SUMMARY AND CONCLUSION

- Isolated of two compounds, 1 and 2.
- Based upon spectral studies, compound 1 was characterized as 2-(1,6a,6b,9,9,12a,14b-heptamethyl 1,2,4a,5,6,6a,6b,7,9,10,11,12,12a,12b,13, 14b-hexadecahydropicen-3-yl)propan-2-yl nonanoate.
- Compound 2 was found to be not pure enough to be characterized.
- Both the compounds were ineffective against breast cancer.
- Petroleum ether and chloroform extracts were effective against breast cancer.

REFERENCES

- Arambewela, L.S.R., Ranatunge, T., 1991. Indole alkaloid from *Tabernaemontana divaricata.* Phytochemistry 30, 1740-1751.

- Bao, M,F., Yan, J.M., Cheng, G.G., Li, X.Y., Liu, Y.P., Li, Y., Cai, X.H., Luo, X.D., 2013. Cytotoxic indole alkaloids from *Tabernaemontana divaricata.* Journal of Natural Products 76, 1406-1412.

- Chaiyana, W., Schripsema, J., Ingkaninan, K., Okonogi, S., 2013. 3'-R/S-hydroxyvoacamine, a potent acetylcholinesterase inhibitor from *Tabernaemontana divaricata.* Phytomedicine 20, 543-548.

- Duarte, R.A., Mello, E.R., Araki, C., Vda, B.S., Siqueira e Silva, D.H., Regasini, L.O., Silva, T.G., de Morais, M.C., Ximenes, V.F., Soares, C.P., 2010. Alkaloids extracted from *Pterogyne nitens* induce apoptosis in malignant breast cell line. Tumor Biology 31, 513-522.

- Elkady, A.I., Abuzinadah, O.A., Baeshen, N.A., Rahmy, T.R., 2012. Differential Control of Growth, Apoptotic Activity, and Gene Expression in Human Breast Cancer Cells by Extracts Derived from Medicinal Herbs *Zingiber officinale.* Journal of Biomedicine and Biotechnology 2012, 1-14.

- Guyton and Hall, Textbook of Medical Physiology, Elsevier saunders, 11th edition, 40-44.

- Hossain, M.A., AL-Raqmi, K.A.L., AL-Mijizy, Z.H., Weli, A.M., Riyamio, Q., 2013. Study of total phenol, flavonoids contents and phytochemical screening of various leaves crude extracts of locally grown *Thymus vulgaris.* Asian Pacific Journal of Tropical Biomedicine 3, 705-710.

○ Julio, E., Díaz-Guerra1, M., Riese, H.H., Alvarez, A., Proenza, R., Fernández, J., 2000. The Cytolytic Effect of a Glycoconjugate Extracted from Corms of Saffron Plant (*Crocus sativus*) on Human Cell Lines in Culture. Planta Medica 66, 157-162.

○ Kam, T.S., Pang, H.S., Choo, Y.M., Komiyama, K., 2004. Biologically active ibogan and vallesamine derivatives from *Tabernaemontana divaricata*. Chemistry & Biodiversity 1, 646-656.

○ Keimei, T., Takashi, K., Hiroki, K., Seok, K.T., Anurada, S., Men, L.T., Conophylline quinone as a new antitumor agent. Jpn. Kokai Tokkyo Koho, assignee. Patent JP 10045763 A 19980217. 17 Jan. 1998.

○ Kundu, N., Campbell, P., Hampton, B., Lin, C.Y., Ma, X.,Ambulos, N., Zhao, X.F., Goloubeva, O., Holt, D., Fulton, A.M., 2012. Antimetastatic activity isolated from *Colocasia esculenta* (taro). Anticancer Drugs 23, 200-211.

○ Lee, A.T.C., Azimahtol, H.L.P., Tan, A.N., 2003. Styrylpyrone Derivative (SPD) induces apoptosis in a caspase-7-dependent manner in the human breast cancer cell line MCF-7. Cancer Cell International 3, 1-8.

○ Masfria., Harahap, U., Nasution, M.P., Ilyas, S., 2013. The activity of *Rhaphidophora pinnta* L. Schott leaf on MCF-7 cell line. Advances in Biological Chemistry 3, 397-402.

○ MCF-7 cells. http://www.mcf7.com (Accessed on 13th Jan. 2014).

○ Mukhram, M.A., Shivakumar, H., Viswanatha, G.L., Rajesh, S., 2012. Anti-fertility effect of flower extracts of *Tabernaemontana divaricata* in rats. Chinese Journal of Natural Medicines 10, 58-62.

○ Orawan, M., De-Eknamkul, W., Umehara, K., Yoshinaga, Y., Miyase, T., Warashina, T., Noguchi, H., 2005. Phenolic Constituents of the Rhizomes of the Thai Medicinal Plant *Belamcanda chinensis* with Proliferative Activity for Two Breast Cancer Cell Lines. Journal of Natural Products 68, 361-364.

○ OECD 423 guidelines. http://ntp.niehs.nih.gov/iccvam/suppdocs/feddocs/oecd/oecd_gl423.pdf (Accessed on 13th Jan. 2014).

○ Pratchayasakul, W., Pongchaidecha, A., Chattipakorn, N., Chattipakorn, S., 2008. Ethnobotany & ethnopharmacology of *Tabernaemontana divaricata*. Indian Journal of Medical Research 127, 317-335.

○ Raj, C.N., Balasubramaniam, A., 2011. Pharmacogostic antimicrobial studies of the leaves of *Tabernaemontana divaricata* R. Pharmacologyonline 2, 1171-1177.

○ Raaman N. 2006. Phytochemical techniques 2, 19-25.

○ Richie, R.C., Swanson, J.O., 2003. Breast Cancer: A Review of the Literature. Journal of Insurance Medicine 35, 85–101.

○ Scambia, G., Ranelletti, F.O., Panici, P.B., De Vincenzo, R., Bonanno, G., Ferrandina, G., Piantelli, M., Bussa, S., Rumi, C., Cianfriglia, M., Quercetin potentiates the effect of adriamycin in a multidrug-resistant MCF-7 human breast-cancer cell line: P-glycoprotein as a possible target. Cancer Chemotherapy Pharmacology 34, 459-464.

○ Sepehr, M.F., Jameie, S.B., Hajijafari, B., 2011. The *Cuscuta kotschyana* effects on breast cancer cells line MCF7. Journal of Medicinal Plants Research 5, 6344-6351.

○ Skehan, P., Storeng, R., Scudiero, D., Monks, A., McMahon, J., Vistica, D., Warren, J.T., Bokesch, H., Kenney, S., Boyd, M.R., 1990. New Colorimetric Cytotoxicity Assay for Anticancer-Drug Screening. Journal of the National Cancer Institute 82, 1107-1112.

○ Surendra, P., Ericka, S., Barry, G., 1997. Curcumin and genistein, plant natural products, show synergistic inhibitory effects on the growth of human breast cancer MCF-7 cells induced by estrogenic pesticides. Biochemical & Biophysical Research Communications 233, 692-696.

○ Valiyari, S., Baradaran, B., Delazar, A., Pasdaran, A., Zare, F., 2012. Dichloromethane and Methanol Extracts of *Scrophularia oxysepala* Induces Apoptosis in MCF-7 Human Breast Cancer Cells. Advanced Pharmaceutical Bulletin 2, 223-231.

YOUR KNOWLEDGE HAS VALUE

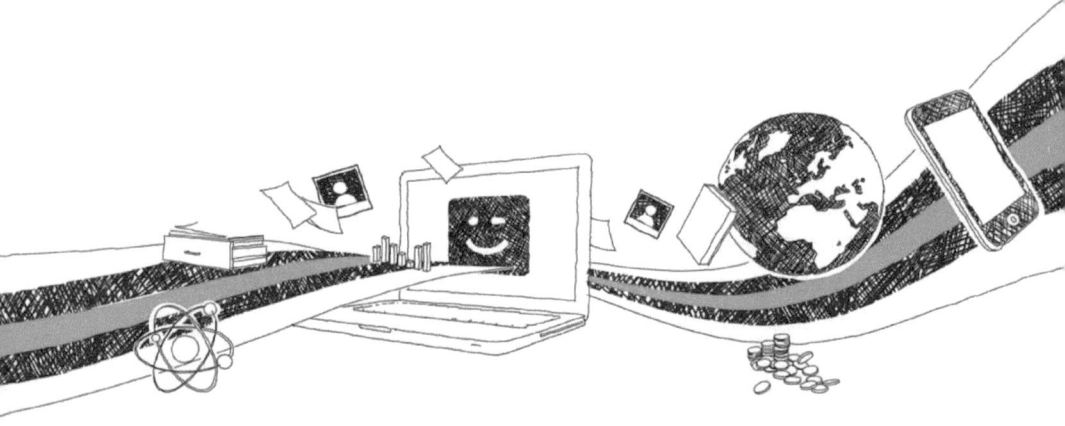

- We will publish your bachelor's and
  master's thesis, essays and papers

- Your own eBook and book -
  sold worldwide in all relevant shops

- Earn money with each sale

Upload your text at www.GRIN.com
and publish for free

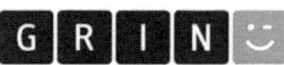